# Test Ride

Christine Holt

ISBN: 0692073698
ISBN-13: 978-0692073698

# DEDICATION

I dedicate this book to my dear family and friends.
Their love and support still overwhelms me, even to this day.
I hope that the love and gratitude that I express in this book
can find a way to all of their hearts. All of their love truly
cradled my heart when I needed it most.

# CONTENTS

# TEST RIDE

# ACKNOWLEDGMENTS

For those in the medical field that had a part in saving my life,
you are amazing and should be proud of what you do every day of your life.
The staff at the rehabilitation center and my amazing team. Your patience
and skill helped me to get back to the life I knew. The writers that guided
me in expressing my thoughts and transferring them to paper and all along
keeping this book truly coming from my heart, that is an art in itself.
I hope that the love and gratitude that I express in this book
can find a way to all of your hearts.

# PROLOGUE

*Hello, this is Christine's sister, just want you to know that she was involved in a horse accident. She had surgery yesterday and is in ICU. The doctor said she should make a full recovery. Her skull was fractured and they had to open it up to relieve pressure. The brain scan looks good. She is sedated till tomorrow sometime. It was a very serious injury and we are very lucky that she pulled through...*

*2 days later -*
*Johnny and I just came down to the hospital and saw her a few minutes. They removed the ventilator, her vitals are good and she squeezed the nurse's hand. She needs to remain very calm and that is why she is still sedated.*

*Following days -*
*The breathing tube is out but she still has a small ventilator to help her if needed. Her eyes are slightly more open, you can tell she's starting to notice things.*

*She is moved into a regular room. She has a feeding tube in her nose and there is still some swelling on the face/eyes but her face is totally intact, the impact was on the right side.*

*There is improvement, she will need to go to rehab for her brain. Even though the brain scan shows the brain being completely fine, she will need work due to the head trauma.*

Why do I have this urge to write about what happened to me? Why can't I let it go? When I walked into work two months after my accident, everyone said I had an amazing recovery. I had escaped without brain damage – truly a miracle.

Why This Urge to Write ...?

Because -
When I hear a helicopter and I look for LifeFlight and I cry ...

Because -
I still want to hug everyone that had a part in that day, in helping me, in helping my family ...

Because -
I feel my head at night, the indention in my skull from where they had to cut the scalp in my emergency operation ...

Because -
I know I am extremely lucky to be alive ...

It must not have been my time to leave everybody. I was meant to stay. My dad must've said "No, leave her there, God. She has to be there for her family, to see her children grow."

I don't know what was the strongest pull, but even though all of my family and friends know what happened to me, they don't know the emotional side of it all - of what I experienced, what I observed and also, of what I learned of love. This was the love that happened while I was lying in ICU, sedated and fighting to live.

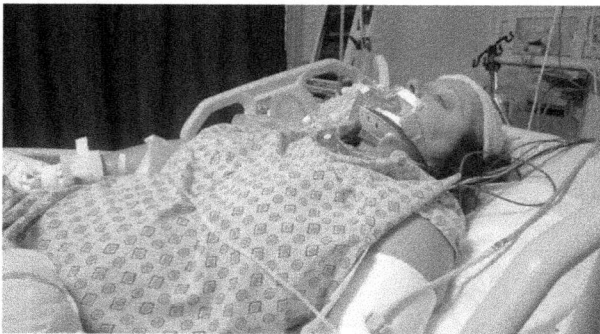

# THE DAY

It was Saturday, October 17, 2015, my husband Johnny's birthday. He was going to go hunting later in the afternoon, but I assured him that I should be back to see him before he went. I was heading out to test ride a horse for the second time. Both Jill, the woman that boarded the horse, and I, agreed that we should take him on a trail ride in the woods, since I had just ridden him in the ring the first time I came out to Jill's farm.

He seemed like a nice horse, a small 12-year old Morgan, who I could tell hadn't been ridden much, but he seemed fine. My 14-year old daughter had even rode him a little the first time we came out.

Jill helped me tighten up my saddle and that was the last thing I remember the day I almost died.

# THE RIDE

Jill heard me say, "Whoa" several times as she walked toward the barn to get her horse. She glanced back to check on me and I was lying on the ground. She rushed to me and cradled my head in her lap as she dialed 9-1-1. Jill told the dispatcher I was snoring loudly, which is a symptom of a concussion. An off-duty EMT, Jamie, heard the 9-1-1 call as she was driving by the barn, and turned around and came to the barn to help.

Thank goodness, she did! She provided comfort and care as the ambulance was on its way. LifeFlight was called and could pick me up four miles down the road at the firehall. From there it would transport me to the hospital 50 miles away – time was of the essence.

I had level two head trauma, as my diagnosis read: Acute right epidural hematoma causing life-threatening brain compression with a complex comminuted open skull fracture on the right side.

I had experienced a focal blunt trauma to my head, so they immediately wheeled me into the operating room for the life-saving epidural hematoma evacuation.

I was told later by an EMT that while I was in the ambulance for those four miles that I almost left them two times. I was shocked to hear this. I knew it was critical to get to the hospital quickly, but had no idea that I was close to death even in the ambulance.

# RELAYING THE NEWS

Jill knew my neighbor across the road and asked her to tell Johnny, that I had just been lifeflighted to the hospital.

Shocked and scared, my husband called his cousin who he was to hunt with and told him the news. Since his cousin's girlfriend knows the Pittsburgh area well, they offered to drive him there. He told our two kids, Clayton, 12 and Autumn, 14 and they got ready. He then called my sister Deb and she grabbed our mother so they could all rush to the hospital.

When they arrived, my husband said it took a while for them to track me down. Since I was brought in by LifeFlight helicopter, I was whisked immediately into surgery - I was in the operating room.

They all waited anxiously for the doctor to appear. My dear mother just sat and prayed, with her strong faith comforting her. They said it seemed like eternity, watching the doctor walk down the hall before beckoning my husband and my sister into his office. The doctor didn't close the door - which was taken as a good sign by Johnny. He first told them that I had made it through the operation fine and was in intensive care.

Then the doctor proceeded to explain the operation in detail. He asked about my general health at the time of this accident. My husband said basically I was not one to sit still, I had a punching bag, a treadmill, and I loved to walk. What the doctor said next was the statement my husband hung on to, "I expect her to have 100% recovery." My husband, (who is not the overly emotional type) and my sister, gave each other a huge hug. This is what started the uniting of family and friends with love while I lay, unaware. I was sedated and not knowing that the next 48 hours was going to be tough on all my loved ones.

# THE WAIT

The next 48 hours were crucial. It was a time when infection or swelling could set in, that I could have trouble. The hospital supplied my husband and sister with the call-in numbers and the passwords so they could check in on me. They drove back home with nothing they could do but wait. Johnny's aunt was outside waiting in front of her house with a big pot of spaghetti which they picked up and they all went to our house to eat and to talk.

For two days, I was kept under heavy sedation and monitored very closely, because my brain needed to be calm to heal. It was a difficult two days for my family. When they came back down to see me, the visitation was limited to an hour at a time, and my heart had to stay at a slow, steady rate. My head was bandaged, I had drainage tubes in my head and a feeding tube was down my throat.

I do not remember my stay in the hospital at all. I asked plenty of questions afterward trying to piece together those ten days of my life that are now gone.

I was visited by many. One faithful friend came during the daytime, in case I came to and was frightened of where I was. Friends from work, and from my life, and family. So many.

After I finally regained consciousness, I was thirsty, and I wanted everyone's drink, some even hid their drinks. Ginger Ale was first on my list – for that was the only pop that I drank, but at that time – I would have taken any of the drinks my family had.

I was showing some signs that gave them hope. Jill came down to visit me and I recognized her, even though I really had only seen her a few times in my life. My brain was working! I knew she was my angel. I was told I followed my husband's voice, as he moved about the room, talking to me.

# OH MY KIDS

I want to cry when I think of how this trauma affected my children. The first day my daughter came in my room but my son couldn't – he hung back. Everyone was worried that I would not recognize them, but I did. Their names came out slowly, but I knew them.

After six days, I was moved into recovery. After that, I had to be moved to a rehabilitation facility of our choice. My sister-in-law and sister took this task. My sister-in-law had been a nurse and had the experience of working with patients with brain trauma. This was a big relief to my husband. They chose a facility which was highly rated and the paperwork was started.

In the meantime, each small step was celebrated. For example, that day I washed my face and brushed my teeth. That was a huge accomplishment and great news to all.

# TEN DAYS LATER

Now I can write directly from my memory.

My husband was walking along beside me and I was so surprised to see him, so I asked him, "Johnny, what are you are doing here?" Then I saw my friend who used to work with me and asked her the same thing, "Bunny, what are you doing here? I haven't seen you for ages!" My sister and another dear friend were there to see me make this encouraging move which was the start of my rehabilitation.

Never mind the fact that I did not question why I was in an ambulance stretcher being wheeled into a strange place.

They put me in the bed and I was looking around, trying to make sense of what was going on. "Where was I?" "Why am I here?" "Johnny, take me home!". They had to decide whether to put in a catheter or I could urinate on my own. My husband turned to me and decided to work with me. I asked what I had to do and he said that I had to go pee in the toilet. And I said, "Oh, I can do that." So that I did! I got up and went to the bathroom!! The nurses clapped and said how good that was. And I couldn't believe going to the bathroom was such an accomplishment. This was the start of my rehabilitation days.

WHY?

I was in wheelchair and had a cast on my arm. "Why?"

"Because you fell off a horse,"

"What horse?" Again, and again those questions came out of my mouth. "You had a bad head injury." "How did that happen? What horse?" My mind could not make sense of this at all. I asked my husband again and again. I had a sacral fracture and a right clavicle fracture (collarbone).

"Take me home, Johnny."
"I can't, insurance company says you have to be in here." "I want to go home to my house and never leave"

"Never go on vacation again?" my father-in-law asked, in disbelief and laughing to himself, and I said "No."

I could not make sense of this, why did I have to be in this hospital room, away from my family, and far away from home? Stuck in a bed, I was supervised and could not move about freely. Every day started at five a.m. with a nurse pricking my arm and then the doctor came in asking me every day what my name is, where I was and what day it was, what is the date and the year.

I was frustrated, confused, and lonely. I had a dear lady in my room that had her third stroke and she talked to me, frustrated that she could not remember and she said she was ready to die. I understood the best that I could at that time, but I knew I was not ready for that myself and for some reason I was in this room in a place far away.

As I look back on my daily schedules I see that they started to give me these my first full day at the rehab, October 28th. Eleven days later, I had spent ten days at the hospital – ten days of my life that I will never remember. Totally gone, I was somewhere else, while my loved ones were home, suffering and having the hardest time, because of me.

I still carry the note I wrote to my husband when I first started to realize the torture he, my kids, and everyone that I loved had gone through.

# REALITY

During each day of my stay at rehab, I wheeled myself into the bathroom, washed my face, and looked at the stranger in the mirror. My shoulder length hair was half gone. I would put my glasses back on and get dressed for the day.

Each day started with a group breakfast, but I didn't want to be there. Everyone had a different situation going on. Some had strokes, some had motorcycle wrecks, and others I can't even remember. I only did the group breakfast for as long as I had to.

I was not feeling friendly. Later, another patient said I kept to myself.

Going home seemed so far away, so I started to draw my calendars.

I could have asked for a calendar from my family – probably even from the rehab - but the fact that I never asked for something so simple was an indication of why I needed to be there.

I drew October and circled the day that I had had the accident and x'ed all the days that I had been in rehab. Then I noticed the official form on the wall, stating my discharge date was Nov. 18. So, I numbered the days I had left. Too many.

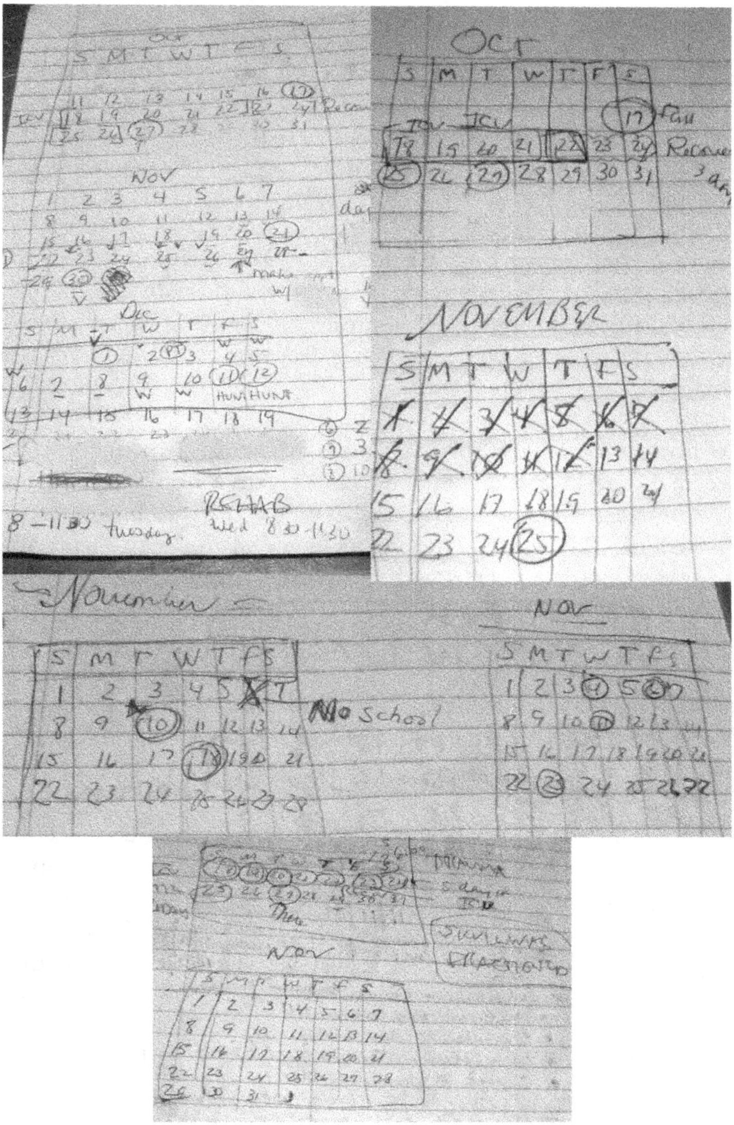
OCT
S M T W T F S
NOVEMBER
S M T W T F S
REHAB
November
S M T W T F S
No School
NOV
S M T W T F S
NOV
S M T W T F S

# VISITORS

One day, my boss and a co-worker walked in. I was so happy to see them both. The company that I worked for sent a huge card, a dear monetary gift and gas/gift cards.

I cried. I cried because of the kindness, generosity and love that was overwhelming to me. Friends came, neighbors and relatives I had not seen for quite some time came in. The cards, the monetary gifts of cash and checks, the gifts of food that were being dropped off at the house – It was overwhelming and I simply cried.

The flowers came. My bedside table was full. I missed my holiday, Halloween. I was known at work for my creative homemade costumes I created every year. Then another co-worker and his wife brought me in the large banner of Halloween Day at work, with all the costumed employees posing for me, some with signs with best wishes and messages for me.

I cried again.

I asked for my computer to be brought in, and I punched the keys in a way that did not indicate that I worked on a computer every day. I had a long way to go ...

My days were like this: physical therapy, speech therapy, lunch and occupational therapy. I needed it all and I needed to work my brain. On my lunch breaks I was able to receive my food in my room - I worked on my brain exercise books that my sister supplied me. In the evenings, I called family or friends if I didn't have visitors. I started my Christmas card writing.

When I was asked how do you make a pizza. I replied - first cheese, pepperoni, sauce then the crust in that order ... more work had to be done.

My release day changed: it was seven days later. "No! I can't do this any longer," was my first thought. I was too removed from home and family, and wanted familiar settings - what we all get used to having and not knowing to appreciate it.

I knew I had to take a driver's test on the computer, pass many tests in my speech therapy and also show how I can get in and out of Johnny's truck before I could go, but I made a decision. I would tell my case manager I want to go home sooner. I gave it some thought and wrote down what i wanted to say to her. I got my appointment with her and made my case. I would do whatever it would take to go home sooner, an additional workout? Whatever I need to, I was mentally ready to go home. She listened and would present this to my team at their weekly meeting.

She came to me and told me the news, they were releasing me earlier. I thanked her and called my husband, to make sure he could get the time off. Then came another surprise. She came into the physical therapy room and said I could go home in 2 days! I wanted to cry with joy! They decided since they don't do any therapies on the weekend, why not let me go home before the weekend!

My husband got off of work in the morning and came down to get me that afternoon. I was in the wheelchair and an arm sling, but I was heading home!!

The ride home was a mixture of things, like questions and taking care of my cravings! "Why doesn't anyone have Halloween decorations up?" I ask my husband on the way home, seemed like they just went to Christmas! A stop to pick up a cup of coffee from my favorite coffee house, along with a cup of my favorite chili and the stop for my prescriptions.

I saw the hard work that my family did - the ramp for my wheelchair, the bed in the living room and a house that was tidy. They have no idea of how much this display of love meant to me.

I had more visitors once I was settled in. My childhood neighbor, who taught me to ride, stopped in and said this is not how I taught you to ride! and at that point I could laugh with her and I totally agreed. She had taught me well. I started riding with her at the age of 12 and after all these years, one horse caught me off-guard.

My mother had Thanksgiving and all came, except for my sister from California but she was there in spirit. I cried again, thanking all of my family for their support. Little did I know at that time I would be shedding more tears in the months of healing that I had yet to do - the mental healing.

My days at home were spent enjoying my family, continuing my physical therapy exercises, and reading all my cards again. I started drawing my Christmas card design and worked with my sister on the wording.

My drawing ended up being a stairway to heaven. It wasn't my first thought, but one morning I woke up with this thought and it seemed the most fitting. I really felt like I was at the bottom of that stairway and I was meant not to climb it at this point of my life.

I must say designing that card with my sister was a special and emotional time, but our end result was perfect for what I was trying to express in my traditional heartfelt Christmas card.

I spent my days while my husband was at work and my kids were at school working on preparing the cards for mail. I always like to add in personal messages and this year I tried to even underline parts of the verses that applied to card recipient. It filled many days.

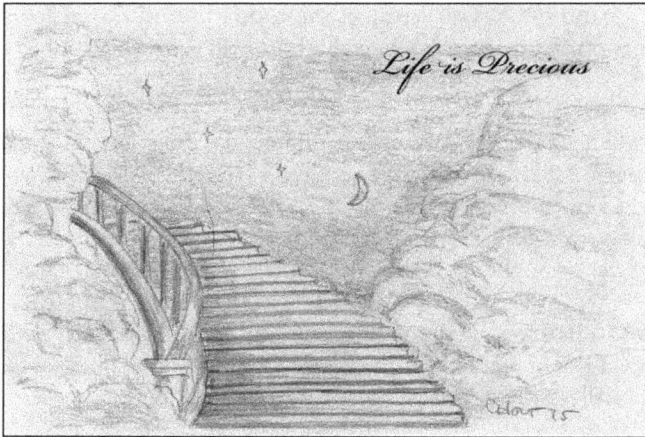

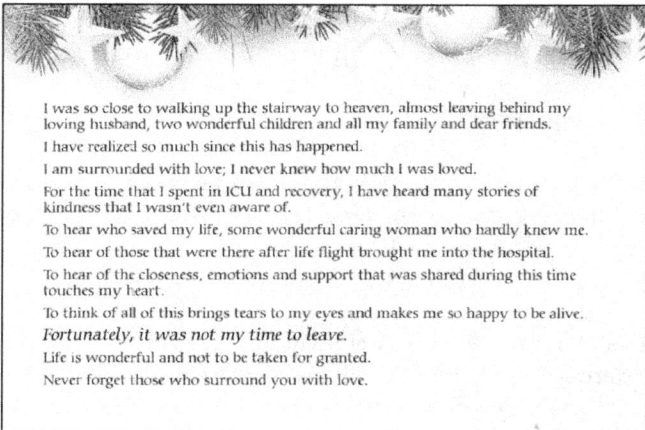

*Life is Precious*

I was so close to walking up the stairway to heaven, almost leaving behind my loving husband, two wonderful children and all my family and dear friends.

I have realized so much since this has happened.

I am surrounded with love; I never knew how much I was loved.

For the time that I spent in ICU and recovery, I have heard many stories of kindness that I wasn't even aware of.

To hear who saved my life, some wonderful caring woman who hardly knew me.

To hear of those that were there after life flight brought me into the hospital.

To hear of the closeness, emotions and support that was shared during this time touches my heart.

To think of all of this brings tears to my eyes and makes me so happy to be alive.

*Fortunately, it was not my time to leave.*

Life is wonderful and not to be taken for granted.

Never forget those who surround you with love.

# TEST RIDE

# I THANKED

I called Jamie, the EMT to thank her for being the first on the scene and she was not even on the clock. I called the ambulance company and praised their staff. I went to the fire hall breakfast so I could meet the other EMTs that treated me.

In the meantime, I had all my follow-up appointments with the neurologist, the orthopedic doctor, and my family doctor. The results were all good. My brother drove us and was there to ask the right questions and to make sure all was covered, being he had been experienced with working with hospitals due to his son's horrifying life-threatening motorcycle accident.

I could try to walk now! I was shaky at first, but it felt great. The first thing I did was package that wheelchair and put it out for pick up. I still could not throw hay bales around, but I could walk to the barn and see my horses!

We weren't sure what kind of Christmas we could give our kids. My husband had talked to them already, because he wasn't sure what we could do. There were presents under that tree come Christmas morning, that were only there because of all the family and friends angels that were around us, once again showing the love that I was so blind to before.

I started to work from home a few hours a day. I walked back into the office three days before Christmas. I was afraid to wait any longer. I wanted to sense if I could do what I did before. I talked, hugged and cried with many. I worked shorter days up until the first of the year, then went back full-time.

My days felt long, but it felt so good to be with my work family again. Then the tears came.

# THE UNEXPECTED...
# AN EMOTIONAL ROLLER COASTER

I was so happy to be alive when I came home and that carried through for the first couple months. Then came the realization of what truly happened hit me. I would be driving home from work and I would think of what my family went through and I would cry.

I would hear a LifeFlight helicopter and I would gaze up at it and cry.

I cried.
I wrote.
I started this book.

I talked, I read. I called my sister-in-law who had worked with those with brain trauma and she said it is about time you go through this! She expected this sooner in me.

I considered going to a support group. I decided against it - It didn't feel right, because I felt like I would not fit in. I was lucky to not have brain damage; it is so common with my kind of injury. I read more and more. I was not crazy for feeling this way, this is normal.

I made a decision – "Let the Ride Go On!

My life had changed. I realized it and came to terms with it. I don't know how others who have gone through a close call with death have handled this, or if they even rode the roller coaster.

I went through a phase of wanting every day to be perfect. Why not? I almost died, life should be perfect, day in and day out. I talked to friends and realized that life is not going to play out like that. Alright, then I am going to just roll with what feelings come my way and act upon what comes over me.

# MY TOUR

I wanted to retrace my days at the hospital. From LifeFlight coming in until I left in the ambulance en-route to the rehab.

The opportunity presented itself in a conversation with an old friend who now works for the hospital network, I mentioned how I would love to trace back those 10 days of my life that will never be a part of my own memory.

She asked and to my surprise it was arranged!

I walked into that hospital, armed with my hospital records and met the man she was able to arrange my visit with. He was a kind man; he asked "What do you want from today?" I said I want to retrace my time there and if I get to meet those that had a part in saving my life, all the better. I still had the continuing need to thank more, to show gratitude and the love I felt, and that I did.

I saw the LifeFlight helicopter pad and control room, the shock trauma room, the operating dept. and my room in ICU. I stood in the waiting room where my family would have been waiting to hear the news. The room where the neurologist would have motioned my husband and sister in to tell them the news that they were on edge to hear. I must say, I was emotionally overwhelmed at that moment and he sensed it and asked if I was OK. "Yes, just taking it all in." I replied.

# SHAKING HANDS AND GIVING HUGS

A nurse that worked with me, I met and hugged. I shook hands with the head of the surgical unit, the Lifeflight control room management, doctors, nurses and so many that he introduced me to and told them why I was there. I learned so many things that day. I learned that my LifeFlight helicopter came from the local airport, my life-saving ride was 16 minutes and most of all, those in the medical field don't get visits from patients like me enough. Everyone I met was so appreciative and thankful for MY words of thanks. What a day! This kind man had people waiting in his office for a meeting, but he introduced me when we rushed back to his office. He spent almost 2 hours with me that day. I sent him a thank you and also one of my Christmas cards.

That kind man had no idea that the time he spent with me left me sitting in my car in their parking lot for a half hour. Overwhelmed with emotion, but all in such a good way.

It is hard for me to describe what a feeling it was to be able to show appreciation to everyone that had a part in saving my life. That kind man helped me recover those ten days that I could not remember.

# BACK IN THE SADDLE

I got back in the saddle after my dear friend Judy and I made ourselves hellhats! She learned of these from Facebook. From a man who created one of these for his wife, who suffered head trauma but he knew would get back in the saddle. It is a riding helmet combined with a western hat brim, and your creativity. He was so generous to share the instructions for free on-line for others to make their own.

Judy gave me a helmet for Christmas, so we spent a day finding our supplies and then another special day making our hats together. What a blast! We posted pictures on-line and I also sent a message and photos to the man to thank him. Once again, how many more can I thank?

Oh, it was good to get back on MY horse. I paused a moment as I lifted the saddle onto his back. The last time I had done such a thing to a horse was the beginning of my book and almost the end of my life. I only hesitated for a few seconds, though, took a deep breath, and continued saddling.

What a great ride that day and we had a few more rides that summer. It was hard to schedule rides and coordinate with our work schedules. My husband wasn't comfortable with me riding alone, which I totally understood. We did meet up with others, some with hellhats of their own, when we could. Life was good.

# GUEST OF HONOR

I walked into the house and my husband said the rehabilitation center had called, and I gave him a look and said "No, I am not going back!" in a laughing manner. It was a call about being selected as a rehab champion of 2015. Another rush of emotion came over me, total disbelief and a huge YES!

It was an annual event that they have. Teams that worked with patients were requested to select patients that they felt worked hard for their recovery. That year they had selected seven recipients. I invited my sister, two dear friends and my 92-year-old mother (who was right by my side every step of the way).

The luncheon ceremony was full of wonderful people, the workers, former patients with their families and friends. We had a nice lunch, official photos taken of the seven recipients and the actual awards ceremony. A member of each patient's team spoke and told of the patient's stay and why they chose them. Then they handed the plaque to the patient.

My speech therapist, Loretta, spoke for me. I laughed as she said everyone that met me knew I wanted to go home! She said that I needed to have everything under control and was lost without it (for those that know me well, that was a fitting statement.) It was her job to help me pull everything together in my brain: from hard brain teasers, reading stories and answering summary questions to figure out the best specials in a grocery store ad. Her speech was wonderful. Then I asked to speak so I could thank everyone and share my hellhat with them.

What a strange feeling it was to walk the halls freely, not in a wheelchair. I saw patients and really felt for them. Being at a rehabilitation center made me see another part of life. It brought me to the ground level of empathy, which, to me, is an amazing bridge of connection to others.

# TWO NURSES AND A PILOT

January 2017

Time passed; I finally watched a documentary about LifeFlight that my husband had told me about. Immediately after watching it, I was on the phone.

I have never met my LifeFlight crew and I may be able to connect to them if I reach out now. After three phone calls, I was able to obtain the head of marketing for LifeFlight contact information. I called and told him my story and desire to meet the crew. I got as far as getting their first names at the hospital tour, but I still hadn't met them. He said he will contact them and see if it can be arranged. It was!

Next thing I knew, I was at the local airport where LifeFlight was stationed and wondered, why I was there? Am I crazy? To relive this again, over a year later? Some would not want to do this, but for me, for who I am, I was there. It was the right thing to do. That settles it, I told myself it will be fine. I waited until the time and gave the marketing director a call. He could not make it due to sickness, but the nurses were in there waiting for me. Ok, here we go.

I met both nurses, the pilot and even a young woman that is in schooling to be a doctor at the hospital trauma dept. that I was in. They were surprised by this request of mine to meet them, to give them each a hug and were so thankful for my visit.

I asked a lot of questions, from what did they know of me before they got on the scene, how long do they spend with the paramedics from the ambulance, what did they do with me in flight?

"Can we go sit in the helicopter," I asked. I found out where each of them sat and how the pilots communicate with the ground crew. I came away with a total respect for those in this field. I sent the Director a thank-you note, a photo of us and also a story he could use on their website.

Mission completed. I felt this was a hard step for me, but it was the last step of my healing process.

# EPILOGUE

It took me over two years to finish this book.

I have read so much about Traumatic Brain Injury (TBI) since then and what I wrote in this book is nothing compared to those that are changed physically and mentally for the rest of their lives. It is a heavy load for their loved ones and their lives are changed also.

This accident changed me in many ways that those close to me may not even realize. The long-lasting effects of head trauma has given me a new perspective. I only take in what is important to me. I don't have to be superwoman anymore. That weekend to-do list I had after a hard week at work was insane, too long and never complete. It is now a thing of the past.

It is not quantity, it is now all quality. I was so driven before, that I think I didn't really spend the time to enjoy life, every moment. We all get caught up in our work, our busy lives and take things for granted. It is a natural thing to do.

I am proud of what I do for a living and I still give my work 100%, because that is who I am. But I am also the person who will sit and wait patiently for the elderly to cross the street and who reads about someone who suffered an injury like mine and reaches out to them. I have acted upon every thought I had along this journey. I am so glad that I made the effort to meet and thank everyone that I could.

I still have something left to do. I am not sure of what it is, but I still have a sense that there is some purpose for me. Maybe it will come soon, maybe later. When I know what it is, I will follow through with it.

# ABOUT THE AUTHOR

Christine continues to write. Something with this traumatic event in her life has brought out a side that she was not even aware existed within. She continues to go with the flow with her pen on both ends, writing and design.